Life Without
NUTS

The Nut-allergy Sufferer's Guide to Safe Eating

Life Without
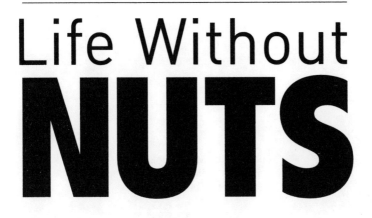

Caroline Jackson

metro

Published by Metro Publishing Ltd,
3 Bramber Court, 2 Bramber Road,
London W14 9PB, England

www.blake.co.uk

First published in paperback in 2004

ISBN 1 84358 082 9

British Library Cataloguing-in-Publication Data:

A catalogue record for this book is available from the British Library.

Design by www.envydesign.co.uk

Printed in Great Britain by Creative Print & Design (Wales) Ltd.

1 3 5 7 9 10 8 6 4 2

Papers used by Metro Publishing are natural, recyclable products made
from wood grown in sustainable forests. The manufacturing processes
conform to the environmental regulations of the country of origin.

Every attempt has been made to contact the relevant copyright-holders,
but some were unobtainable. We would be grateful if the appropriate
people could contact us.

Acknowledgements

Many thanks to David Reading of The Anaphylaxis Campaign for all his help and advice.

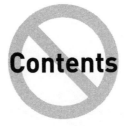

Contents

PART TWO – THE RECIPES

Introduction

*L*ife Without Nuts is a book that aims to make the life of the nut-allergy sufferer that bit more enjoyable. It is not going to take away the necessity for constant vigilance; being very aware of what makes up the food you are eating is the most important lesson the nut-allergy sufferer can learn. It could literally save your life. Instead, this book looks at the sorts of food that often contain nuts, and attempts to suggest alternatives, or nut-free versions, so that you can play safe without feeling left out.

In addition to this, I have collated some essential information about nut allergies, which I hope will be helpful to those who discover that a friend or relative suffers from the condition, or for new parents who have a child who is allergic to nuts. It goes without saying, of course, that, if you or your child is displaying even the mildest signs of nut allergy, you must speak to your doctor immediately. He or she will advise you on the best course of action, and will explain to you the treatments available. There are also a number of organisations that provide advice and support to allergy sufferers; a list of these is supplied at the back of this book.

A final word of advice: everybody is different. Some people are allergic to certain nuts, and other people aren't. There are ways of testing what you are allergic to, and we will discuss these later in the book. The recipes in this book avoid all the major allergens, but that does not mean that you should be blasé when preparing the food. This is especially the case that you should be careful with shop-bought sauces and other products. Always read the labels very carefully, and if you are in any doubt at all – ask! That way you can be sure of preparing these delicious recipes in a way that is safe for you.

PART ONE –
The Basics

What is Nut Allergy?

Allergies are immune responses to substances, or allergens, to which the body has become hypersensitive. There are many types of allergy: hay fever is an allergic response to pollen; and people can develop allergic responses to all sorts of food – shellfish or milk, for example.

Nut allergy is the most serious form of food allergy. It currently affects about 1.3 per cent of the population, and the bad news is that it's on the increase. No one quite knows why this should be so, but it is thought that it is partially due to the fact that additional people are being exposed to peanuts in particular, as they are being used more and more in the preparation and manufacture of food. On top of that, the age of onset of peanut allergy appears to be reducing, and an accelerating number of infants are being diagnosed with it.

Whereas certain allergies have a tendency to be outgrown, this appears to be less likely with nut allergy. Only about 20 per cent of childhood sufferers grow out of their allergy to peanuts.

Responses to the allergens vary from person to person. Some people might eat a small quantity of nut and experience only a mild swelling around the lips. Others will experience a severe allergic response which results in the swelling of tissues in the body and, if the throat is involved, possibly asphyxiation. This extreme response is called anaphylaxis. Anaphylactic responses do not only come from nuts, but, whatever the allergen, they are extremely dangerous and sometimes fatal. In the UK alone, six known deaths occur every year as a result of peanut or nut anaphylaxis, although other fatalities may be wrongly attributed to other causes. Even if symptoms triggered by nuts are apparently mild, they must be taken seriously. A subsequent reaction may be more severe.

What are the Symptoms?

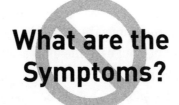

The symptoms of nut allergy are quite diverse, and they can become more or less severe each time they occur. The following are all possible symptoms which may occur when exposed to an allergen, and you may experience one or more of them:

- Sneezing
- Swelling of the face, lips, tongue, throat or any other part of the body
- A general flushing of the skin
- A sense of fear
- Difficulty in breathing and talking, and sudden wheezing
- Asthma attacks in asthmatics
- An itchy skin rash, sometimes called 'nettlerash'
- Stomach cramps
- Vomiting

- Low blood pressure, leading to faintness and sometimes unconsciousness
- Severe anaphylactic shock causing obstruction to breathing or extremely low blood pressure

These symptoms often appear within seconds or minutes of being exposed to nuts, but even the most severe reactions may appear or reappear several hours later.

All of these symptoms should be taken seriously, but anaphylactic shock is the most alarming and indeed the most dangerous. When the allergen enters the blood stream, it triggers a massive release of the chemical histamine, along with other chemicals. This causes a widening of the blood vessels, which can lead to blood pressure dramatically and severely lowering, and the constriction of air passages in the lungs. In severe cases this leads to asphyxiation. Please note, however, that anaphylactic shock is not common. In children, it is particularly rare. Impaired breathing caused by asthma or swelling is more common and this is serious in itself.

How are Nut Allergies Diagnosed and Treated?

It might seem obvious, but it is worth saying: the best treatment for nut allergies is to avoid the allergen in the first place. If you don't come into contact with nuts, you can't react to them and so, as I've said before, it is essential that the nut-allergy sufferer pays constant attention to the constituent parts of the foods that he or she eats.

But, of course, sometimes things go wrong. When a severe reaction occurs to the consumption of nuts or nut-related products, it must always be treated as an emergency. If it is not treated immediately, it can be fatal.

The recommended treatment for a severe allergic reaction is the administering of an adrenaline injection (also known by its official name Epinephrine). The two most common adrenaline injections go under the brand names of EpiPen and Anapen. If you are prescribed one, carry it at all times. (Your doctor will prescribe these injections, and there are 'practice pens' you can use to get the hang of administering them.) The adrenaline works by constricting blood vessels which can swell and leak during anaphylactic shock, relaxing muscles in the lungs, stimulating the heart beat and reducing swelling on the face.

Immediately a serious reaction is suspected, this is what you must do:

- Immediately administer an adrenaline injection
- Call an ambulance
- If there is no visible improvement after 5–10 minutes, and the ambulance has not arrived, administer a second injection, if available

It is important to call an ambulance. The patient will probably need to be admitted to hospital where further drugs, such as antihistamine or corticosteroid, will be administered.

If you suffer even a mild allergic reaction, and you are unsure what caused it, you must get tested. There are three main ways of testing for allergies. These are blood tests, skin-prick tests and patch tests. If you suspect that you are allergic to something – not just nuts – your doctor will advise one of these tests.

What Foods Do
I Need to Avoid?

Allergies can be caused by a wide range of foods. The most common allergens which come under the blanket term 'nut allergy' are tree nuts and peanuts (actually a type of legume). If you are a nut-allergy sufferer, you may be allergic to a greater or lesser extent to one or more of these types of nut. The following is a list of nuts that are commonly advised to be avoided if you are a nut-allergy sufferer:

- **Peanuts** (also known as **groundnuts, monkey nuts** and **earth nuts)**
- **Almonds** (including almond essence)
- **Brazil nuts**
- **Cashew nuts**
- **Chob nuts**
- **Macadamia nuts**
- **Pecan nuts**
- **Pistachio nuts**

- **Walnuts**
- **Arachis oil** (an extract of peanuts often found in pharmaceutical products)

Chestnuts, pine nuts and coconuts are not commonly regarded as causing nut allergy but some sufferers may react to them, so caution is advisable. In fact, if you are allergic to one kind of nut, doctors will often advise you to avoid other nuts. It may be that you are allergic only to peanuts, for example, in which case other nut products will not be problematic. You can only be sure of this, though, by taking an allergy test. *Cooking nuts does not reduce their allergenicity.*

None of the recipes in this book contains any of the above foods.

OILS

Nuts, especially peanuts, are used to make cooking oils. Generally speaking, the nut oils are refined, and research into peanut oils has shown that they pose little or no threat to the nut-allergy sufferer. However, you might feel safer avoiding even refined nut oils – it is not a good area for experimentation. Unrefined nut oil is dangerous.

Vegetable oil is a mixture of various oils, and may contain peanut oils. Again, these are generally refined, but you have no way of being sure.

Sesame oil and walnut oil should be avoided, because they are generally unrefined.

All the recipes in this book use sunflower oil or olive oil, both of which are usually safe to the nut-allergy sufferer.

COCONUTS

Very few people who suffer from nut allergies have a problem with coconuts, but instances have been recorded. For safety's sake, none of the recipes in this book contains coconut.

NUTMEG

Nutmeg is not a nut. Although some people are allergic to it, it is not generally a problem for nut-allergy sufferers.

OTHER LEGUMES

As we have already learned, peanuts are classed as legumes. There is no reason to avoid other legumes such as peas, lentils and beans unless you suspect you are allergic to them.

Allergy Labelling

It is vitally important that you learn to read the labels of any food you are going to put in your mouth or any cream or lotion you are going to put on your skin.

Unfortunately, the regulations controlling food labelling are not as clear or stringent as they might be. Currently, in the UK, the ingredients of pre-packaged food must be listed in descending order of quantity. In Autumn 2003, the law changed concerning food labelling – all major allergenic ingredients now have to be listed on food packaging. However, the change will not be fully effective until 2005.

Most food manufacturers are responsible, and will say on the packaging 'May contain traces of nuts'. This is particularly important where nut-free foods are prepared on the same production line as foods that do contain nuts. The risk of cross-contamination may be small, but you should be aware of it.

There is some concern that food manufacturers are

over-using the 'May contain traces of nuts' label in order to cover their backs. From the point of view of the nut-allergy sufferer, this can be annoying – but nevertheless better safe than sorry.

The following is a list of points to remember when scrutinising labels:

- Always do it!
- Just because a product does not say 'May contain traces of nuts', it does not mean it doesn't contain any. Always read the product's ingredients carefully.
- If you are allergic to peanuts, remember that they can also be called groundnuts, monkey nuts and earth nuts.
- Just because you have safely eaten a product potentially at risk from cross-contamination once, it doesn't mean you should do it again. It may have avoided cross-contamination on one occasion, but it won't necessarily do so in the future.
- Certain pharmaceutical products contain arachis oil. This is derived from peanuts but will probably be refined and may well be safe to use.
- If you are at all concerned about a particular food, contact the manufacturer to check it out. If you are still concerned, *don't eat it*.

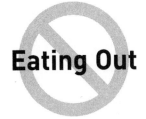

Eating Out

Restaurants are under no obligation to list the ingredients of the food they serve, and this can put the food-allergy sufferer in a very dangerous position. If you are at all unsure about a particular meal, question the waiter or waitress very carefully about your selection. If you are not satisfied by their response, ask to speak to the manager, and, if you are still not satisfied, go and eat somewhere else. You might find it a good idea to call the restaurant in advance to make sure that they are 'allergy aware'.

Certain cuisines use nuts more than others: you should avoid Chinese, Indian and Thai restaurants, as well as anywhere serving other Eastern cuisines. Even if a particular dish does not contain nuts, they are so widely used in these types of cooking that the danger of cross-contamination is ever-present. In this book you will find recipes for Chinese, Indian and Thai foods so that you don't feel left out!

The problem of eating out is a main reason why you should

be very open with your friends and family about your nut allergy – if everybody knows you have a problem with Indian food, they won't keep suggesting that you go out for a curry ...

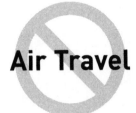

Air Travel

There are a number of reasons why air travel can cause problems for the nut-allergy sufferer. Most obvious is the problem of the food served. Although some airlines will seek to ensure that, on request, a nut-free meal will be available, mistakes can be made, so do be careful. The best option is to take your own food whenever possible.

More problematic is the tendency to serve peanuts as snacks to go with drinks. You can, of course, decline them, but there is concern that remnants of peanut dust can stay on the tables and around the seats. It is advised that nut-allergy sufferers take wet wipes to clean the area where they are sitting, especially the table.

Finally, since September 11, airlines have cracked down on the implements that are allowed to be taken on board, and so some nut-allergy sufferers have experienced difficulties in taking their adrenaline injections on to the airplane. You are advised to do the following to ensure that this is not a problem:

- Contact the airline in advance to warn them that you will need to take your injection kit on to the plane.
- Arrange a note from your doctor to say that you are severely allergic and need to carry your injection with you at all times.
- Mention the fact that you are carrying an injection with you when you check in.
- Make sure that you can demonstrate that you are keeping the injection in a secure place where it cannot be accessed by other passengers.
- Some airlines will insist on keeping the injection for you in a safe place. If this is the case, make sure that the airline staff and your neighbouring passengers are aware of your allergy, know what the symptoms are and how to administer the injection if necessary.

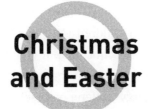

Christmas and Easter

Christmas can be a difficult time for the nut-allergy sufferer. So many of the foods we eat at this time of the year can be dangerous, and so it is important to be extra vigilant. You will find a recipe in this book for a nut-free Christmas cake, and some supermarkets now stock nut-free Christmas puddings and mince pies (and you can order them online at www.itsnutsfree.com). But the problems don't stop there. Here is a list of some of the foods of which you need to be careful when you are planning the Christmas feast. Not all of them necessarily contain nuts, but they very well may do, so do please be careful:

- Christmas pudding
- Christmas cake (see page 48 for an alternative)
- Mince pies
- Pre-dinner snacks (see pages 23–34 for alternatives)
- Nut roasts

- Stuffing
- Chocolates
- Biscuits
- Ice cream

Easter is a time when children (and adults!) are traditionally given large quantities of chocolate. If you are giving an Easter gift to a nut-allergy sufferer, do make sure it is nut-free; and, if you are a nut-allergy sufferer yourself, be extra careful to check that the chocolate you are eating is nut-free. If in doubt, don't eat it.

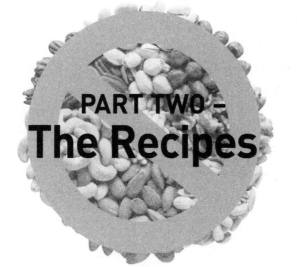

PART TWO –
The Recipes

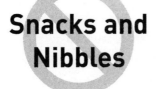

Snacks and Nibbles

For the nut-allergy sufferer, snacks and nibbles can be a nightmare. Not only is no drinks party complete without the ever-present bowl of peanuts, but it's also impossible to tell whether any other pre-packaged snacks – be they crisps, biscuits or whatever – contain traces of nuts or have been prepared in a factory where nuts are used. Clearly it's not a risk you can take.

In this chapter, you will find ten recipes for nibbles that are perfectly safe for the nut-allergy sufferer to eat. They are also a lot more exciting than the standard drinks party fare you're likely to come across – so you can turn the problem of your allergy into an excuse for eating much tastier food!

Aubergine Caviar

SERVES 8

4 large aubergines
½ teaspoon cumin seeds, crushed
1 large garlic clove, very finely chopped
extra virgin olive oil
juice of 3 lemons
1 tablespoon parsley, chopped
salt and freshly ground black pepper

Preheat the oven to 240°C/Gas Mark 9. Place the aubergines on a tray, pop them in the oven and cook until they are soft inside – this should take 45 minutes to an hour. Cut the aubergines in half lengthways, then scoop out the mushy insides. Add the cumin, garlic, lemon juice, parsley and seasoning, then add enough olive oil to make a loose paste. This is good served with fresh bread, or as a dip with raw vegetable crudités.

Black Olive Tapenade

SERVES 8

300g pitted black olives
1 large garlic glove
1 tin anchovy fillets in olive oil
1 teaspoon Dijon mustard
extra virgin olive oil
lemon juice to taste
salt and freshly ground black pepper

Place the olives, garlic, anchovy fillets (including their oil) and mustard in a food processor. Whizz until roughly chopped. Season well, then add the olive oil and lemon juice to taste. This is very good served on pieces of hot, thin toast.

Your Kind of Olives

You can buy a huge range of olives in supermarkets nowadays. Some have been flavoured, some haven't, but why not buy a batch of your favourite and flavour them yourself? All you need to do is place them in a bowl and season them with your favourite flavours. Try to use dried herbs if you can, because that way the olives will keep for longer. Make up your own ingredients, or use three or four of the following:

any dried herb – oregano, thyme, sage or mixed herbs
    are all good
crumbled dried bay leaves
dried chillies
cumin seeds
crushed coriander seeds
fennel seeds
finely chopped garlic
a few sprigs of fresh rosemary
freshly ground black pepper

Place the olives in a jam jar, cover with the best olive oil you can get and store until you're ready to eat them.

Home-made Pâté

400g chicken livers
150g butter
75g double cream

Melt 70g of the butter in a large saucepan. When it is hot and bubbling, add the chicken livers and let them brown quickly on both sides. You want the insides to remain slightly pink. Add the livers, their cooking butter and 30g of the remaining butter to a food processor and blitz till smooth. Add the cream and blitz again.

Pour the mixture into a shallow bowl, and leave in the fridge to set for 30 minutes. Melt the remaining butter, pour on top of the pâté and leave to set in the fridge for a couple of hours. Serve with hot toast.

The pâté will keep for a couple of days.

Home-made Crisps

There is no reason at all why you should limit yourself simply to making potato crisps. Other root vegetables make a great variety. Parsnips are great, and so is beetroot. Choose the vegetables you want to use, peel them, then slice them as thinly as you possibly can. Plunge the slices into cold water, then dry them thoroughly using a clean tea towel. Fry them in a deep-fat fryer until they are golden, drain them on plenty of kitchen towel and sprinkle with sea salt.

Selection of Dips
with Crudités

The crudités are up to you! Raw vegetables are very good – try carrots, cauliflower, courgettes and cucumber – or you could use Italian breadsticks. You could serve the Aubergine Caviar (page 24), or the Black Olive Tapenade (page 25), but here are three more fabulous dips you can easily make at home.

Smoked Mackerel Pâté

SERVES 8

2 smoked mackerel, skinned and flesh
    removed from the bones
100g cottage cheese
150ml Greek yogurt
juice of 1 lemon
grated nutmeg
salt and freshly ground black pepper

Place the fish, cottage cheese and yogurt in a liquidiser with most of the lemon juice. Blend until smooth. Transfer the mixture to a bowl, then season and add a little more lemon juice if you think it needs it. Chill well before serving.

Aioli

SERVES 8

2 garlic cloves, finely chopped
2 egg yolks
1 teaspoon Dijon mustard
1 teaspoon white wine vinegar
250ml olive oil
salt and freshly ground black pepper

Put the garlic, egg yolks, mustard and vinegar in a bowl, and season well. Whisking constantly, add the oil drop by drop and then, very gradually, in a steady trickle until the aioli is good and thick. You can do this in a food processor.

Cream Cheese and Herb Dip

SERVES 8

2 large tubs Philadelphia cheese
2 or 3 tablespoons chopped fresh herbs

Choose whichever herbs take your fancy, and mix them well with the cheese.

Cheese Straws

SERVES 8

350g plain flour
200g butter
40g Parmesan, grated
pinch of cayenne pepper
1 egg, beaten
salt and freshly ground black pepper

Preheat the oven to 375°C/Gas Mark 5. Rub the butter into the flour so that it resembles breadcrumbs. Add the cheese, cayenne pepper and seasoning, and then bind the mixture together with the egg yolk, adding cold water teaspoon by teaspoon if you think it necessary. Roll the pastry out, cut into strips and bake on a well-greased baking tray until the straws are cooked and golden.

Sausage Rolls

SERVES 8

400g sausage meat
1 onion
1 teaspoon dried thyme
1 teaspoon dried sage
400g puff pastry
1 egg, beaten

Preheat the oven to 425°C/Gas Mark 7. Mix the sausage meat, onion and herbs in a bowl. Roll out the puff pastry as thin as you can into a large rectangle. Cut the rectangle into three strips. Divide the sausage meat into three, then shape each portion into a roll the same length as the pastry.

Place one sausage-meat roll on to a pastry strip, then moisten one edge of the pastry with the beaten egg. Fold the pastry over, seal it tightly, then turn the whole thing over so that it is sitting on the sealed edge. Repeat for each strip of pastry. Cut each roll into 5cm pieces, prong with a fork, then brush with egg. Place on a baking sheet and bake for about 20 minutes until golden.

Guacamole

SERVES 8

4 large ripe avocados
juice of 2 lemons
4 large tomatoes, skinned, seeded and finely chopped
1 onion, very finely chopped
2 large garlic cloves, very finely chopped
1 teaspoon medium chilli powder
salt and freshly ground black pepper

Stone, peel and finely chop the avocados, then put them in a bowl with the lemon juice to stop them discolouring. Add the remaining ingredients, season well, cover and keep in a cool place until you are ready to use it.

Cream Cheese and Smoked Salmon Canapés

SERVES 8

2 large tubs Philadelphia cheese
200g smoked salmon, finely chopped
a few water biscuits, broken into bite-sized pieces
salt and freshly ground black pepper

Mix the cheese and the salmon, then season well. Serve generously on the pieces of water biscuit (or any other base you care to choose).

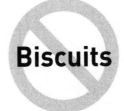

Biscuits

If you have a nut allergy, you really do need to be careful about biscuits. A lot of them contain peanuts, but the real problem lies in the fact that those that don't are often made in the same factories as those that do. Of course, many are perfectly safe, but if you want to be extra sure – and eat much nicer biscuits into the bargain – why not try some of these. And remember: biscuits are really, really easy to make, and home-made ones taste a hundred times nicer than anything you can buy.

Shortbread

MAKES 15–20 BISCUITS

110g butter
60g caster sugar, plus a little extra for dusting
175g plain flour

In a food processor or by hand, thoroughly beat together the butter and sugar, then add the flour and continue beating. Roll the dough out until it is about 3mm thick, then cut out the biscuits using a 7.5cm cutter. Place on a greased baking tray and bake for about 30 minutes. Cool on a wire rack and dust with the extra sugar.

Nut-free Brownies

MAKES 15–20 BISCUITS

100g butter

50g cooking chocolate

2 eggs, beaten

220g caster sugar

50g plain flour

1 teaspoon baking powder

100g raisins

Preheat the oven to 180°C/Gas Mark 4. Grease a deep 20x30cm baking tin and then line it with greaseproof paper. You need a rim of paper about 5cm deep around the tray.

Melt the chocolate and the butter in a glass bowl over a saucepan of boiling water. Remove from the heat, add all the other ingredients and spread the mixture into the tin. Bake for about 30 minutes until a knife inserted in the mixture comes away clean. Leave it to cool and firm up for about 15 minutes, then divide into 15–20 biscuits.

Gingernuts

MAKES ABOUT 15 BISCUITS

100g self-raising flour
1 teaspoon ground ginger
1 teaspoon bicarbonate of soda
40g granulated sugar
50g butter
2 tablespoons golden syrup

Preheat the oven to 190°C/Gas Mark 5. Mix together the flour, ginger, bicarbonate of soda and sugar in a bowl, then lightly rub in the butter until the mixture resembles breadcrumbs. Add the syrup and mix well together.

Divide the mixture into about 15 pieces, then roll each piece into a little ball. Place the balls on a lightly greased baking sheet – leaving plenty of space around each one – and press down slightly to flatten the top of each ball. Bake for about 15 minutes and cool on a wire rack before eating or storing.

Brandy Snaps

MAKES LOTS OF BRANDY SNAPS!

110g flour
110g butter
110g sugar
110g golden syrup
2 teaspoons ground ginger
juice of ½ lemon

Preheat the oven to 190°C/Gas Mark 5. Melt the sugar, butter and syrup together in a saucepan, then add the ginger and lemon. Place teaspoonfuls of the mixture on to a well-greased baking tin and bake until golden brown. Leave to cool for a few moments, then, while still malleable, roll the brandy snaps round the thick handle of a wooden spoon. Leave to cool, then eat – filled with whipped cream if you fancy it.

Easter Biscuits

MAKES ABOUT 15 BISCUITS

225g plain flour
110g butter
grated rind of ½ lemon
110g caster sugar
½ teaspoon baking powder
50g currants
1 large egg, beaten

Preheat the oven to 180°C/Gas Mark 4. Rub the butter and flour together until it resembles breadcrumbs. Add the lemon zest, sugar, baking powder and currants. Mix together with enough egg to create a soft dough. Roll out to a thickness of about ½cm, then use a round cutter to cut out the biscuits. Place on a greased baking tray and bake for about 20 minutes.

Oat Crunchies

MAKES ABOUT 10 BISCUITS

110g porridge oats
75g demerara sugar
110g butter

Preheat the oven to 190°C/Gas Mark 5. Grease a 30x20cm shallow baking tin. Mix the oats and the sugar in a bowl, then gently melt the butter. Add the butter to the oat and sugar mix, and mix until thoroughly combined. Tip the mixture into the tin and bake for about 15 minutes until just golden.

Remove from the oven, and cut the biscuits into portions. Leave in the tin until quite cold, then store (or, more likely, eat!).

Digestive Biscuits

MAKES ABOUT 10 BISCUITS

1 tablespoon granulated sugar

110g plain flour

¼ teaspoon salt

¼ teaspoon bicarbonate of soda

75g butter

110g oatmeal

1 tablespoon milk

Preheat the oven to 180°C/Gas Mark 4. Combine the sugar, flour, salt and bicarbonate of soda and rub in the butter till it resembles breadcrumbs. Mix in the oatmeal, then add the milk and combine to form a soft dough. Roll it out thinly, then use a circular cutter to cut the biscuits. Bake for about 20 minutes until crisp and golden.

Chocolate Valentines

MAKES ABOUT 10 BISCUITS

200g plain flour
110g butter
85g caster sugar
1 egg white
handful of chocolate buttons

Preheat the oven to 150°C/Gas Mark 2. Lightly grease a baking tray. In a food processor or by hand, beat the butter and sugar together until pale. Add the flour and mix well until you have a soft dough. Roll out the dough quite thinly, then, using a heart-shaped cutter, cut out the biscuits.

Brush the edge of the biscuits with egg white and place a chocolate button in the middle. Lay another heart on top and press the edges together so that the biscuit is well sealed. Bake for about 35 minutes, and leave to cool on a wire rack before eating.

Choc-oat Biscuits

MAKES ABOUT 60 BISCUITS

115g plain flour
½ teaspoon bicarbonate of soda
¼ teaspoon baking powder
¼ teaspoon salt
115g soft butter
115g caster sugar
100g demerara sugar
1 egg
½ teaspoon vanilla extract
85g porridge oats
150g plain chocolate chips

Preheat the oven to 180°C/Gas 4. Lightly grease about four baking trays. Combine the flour, bicarbonate of soda, baking powder and salt. In a food processor, beat the butter, caster sugar and demerara sugar well. Add the egg and vanilla extract and continue beating.

Add the flour mixture, and gently fold it in until well combined. Stir in the porridge oats and chocolate chips, mixing well.

Use a teaspoon to place heaped blobs of the crumbly mixture on the baking sheets. Leave a little space around each one, as the biscuits will spread. Bake for about 15 minutes, then let the biscuits cool on a wire rack.

Lemon Treats

MAKES 10–12 BISCUITS

220g plain flour
50g icing sugar, plus a little extra for dusting
¼ teaspoon salt
170g cold butter
1 teaspoon very cold water
4 eggs
450g caster sugar
30g plain flour
½ teaspoon baking powder
grated rind of ½ lemon
juice of 2 large lemons

Preheat the oven to 180°C/Gas Mark 4. Mix the flour, icing sugar and salt in a bowl, then rub in the butter until it resembles breadcrumbs. Add the water and mix until it forms a ball. Gently press the mixture into a 30x20cm baking dish. Bake for about 15 minutes until golden brown. Remove from the oven and allow to cool slightly.

In a food processor, mix together the remaining ingredients. Pour the mixture over the cooled base, then return the whole thing to the oven for a further 20–25 minutes. Allow to cool before dusting with icing sugar and cutting into squares.

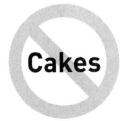

Cakes

Cakes, like biscuits, can be a nightmare for the nut-allergy sufferer. So many of them contain nuts that they are often all simply struck off the list of allowable foods. Here are ten recipes for delicious cakes that are totally safe to eat – starting with a traditional, nut-free Christmas cake, so that you don't have to feel left out every December!

Nut-free Christmas Cake

450g currants

175g sultanas

175g raisins

100g glacé cherries

4 tablespoons brandy

225g plain flour

½ teaspoon salt

¼ teaspoon freshly grated nutmeg

½ teaspoon ground mixed spice

225g unsalted butter

225g demerara sugar

4 eggs

1 tablespoon black treacle

grated zest of 1 lemon

grated zest of 1 orange

To decorate:

2 tablespoons apricot jam (Please note: If you suffer from an allergy to almonds, you might have an apricot intolerance, in which case any jam you can eat will do.)

whole glacé fruits of your choice

The day before you make the cake, place the currants, sultanas, raisins and cherries in a bowl, and soak with the brandy. Cover and leave overnight.

Preheat the oven to 140°C/Gas Mark 1. Grease a 20cm cake tin, and line it with greaseproof paper.

Sift together the flour, salt, nutmeg and mixed spice in a

large mixing bowl. In a food processor, thoroughly beat together the butter and sugar. You may need to stop the mixer now and then to push the mix down the sides of the bowl. Make sure it is very well mixed and pale. Now beat the eggs and add them to the mixture very slowly – a tablespoon at a time – mixing well all the time.

Fold in the flour and spices, and then stir in the fruit and brandy, the treacle and the orange and lemon zest.

Transfer the mixture to the cake tin, then over it place a circle of greaseproof paper, into the centre of which you have cut a small hole about 3cm in diameter. Bake the cake for 4½ hours.

When it is cooked, remove from the tin and allow to cool on a wire rack. When quite cold, you can decorate the cake. Mix the apricot jam with a tablespoon of water, and heat very gently till it is melted and liquid. Use a pastry brush to paint the top of the cake with the jam, and then decorate with the glacé fruits, using more jam to stick them on if necessary. Coat the finished cake with another layer of jam, and store in an airtight container until ready to eat.

Chocolate Cake

115g cooking chocolate

275ml milk

200g demerara sugar

1 egg yolk

250g plain flour

1 teaspoon bicarbonate of soda

½ teaspoon salt

150g butter

250g caster sugar

3 eggs

1 teaspoon vanilla extract

For the icing:

225g cooking chocolate

¼ teaspoon salt

175ml crème fraîche

Preheat the oven to 180°C/Gas Mark 4. Line two 20cm cake tins with greaseproof paper.

Place the chocolate, one third of the milk, the demerara sugar and the egg yolk into a glass bowl. Cook until smooth over a saucepan of boiling water.

Sift the flour, bicarbonate of soda and salt into a bowl.

Cream the butter and sugar together in a food processor, then beat in the whole eggs, one at a time. Stir in the vanilla extract and the remaining milk.

Gently fold the flour mixture into the butter mix until it is well combined. Add the chocolate mixture and fold until just combined. Divide the mixture equally between the two cake tins and bake for about 40 minutes, or until a skewer inserted into the cakes comes away clean. Remove the cakes from the tins and leave to cool on a wire rack.

To make the icing, melt the chocolate in a glass bowl set over a pan of hot water. Remove from the heat and stir in the salt and crème fraîche. Leave it to cool slightly before spreading one third of the icing on one of the cake layers. Place the second layer on top, and spread the remaining icing over the top and sides.

Carrot Cake

225g plain flour

225g sugar

½ teaspoon bicarbonate of soda

½ teaspoon baking powder

½ teaspoon cinnamon

2 eggs

150ml sunflower oil

110g carrot, grated

Preheat the oven to 180°C/Gas Mark 4. Sieve together the flour, bicarbonate of soda, baking powder and cinnamon into a large bowl. Add the sugar. Beat together the eggs and the sunflower oil, and add to the dry ingredients. Stir in the grated carrot and mix well. Transfer to a well-greased loaf tin and bake for 40 minutes, or until a skewer inserted into the cake comes away clean.

Ginger Cake

170g plain flour

2 teaspoons baking powder

½ teaspoon salt

2 teaspoons ground ginger

2 teaspoons ground cinnamon

1 teaspoon ground cloves

¼ teaspoon grated nutmeg

2 eggs

220g caster sugar

250ml double cream

1 teaspoon vanilla extract

Preheat the oven to 180°C/Gas Mark 4. Grease a 20cm square baking tin.

Sift together the flour, baking powder, salt, ginger, cinnamon, cloves and nutmeg. In a food processor, beat together the eggs and sugar until pale. Add the cream and vanilla extract, and mix well. Fold in the dry ingredients until very well combined, then pour the mixture into the tin. Bake for about 40 minutes, until springy. Let the cake cool for 10 minutes or so before cutting into squares.

Madeira Cake

225g soft butter
225g caster sugar
grated zest of 1 lemon
1 teaspoon vanilla extract
4 eggs
225g plain flour
1 teaspoon baking powder

Preheat the oven to 170°C/Gas Mark 3. Grease a 20x15cm loaf tin. In a food processor, beat together the butter and sugar. Stir in the lemon zest and vanilla extract. Add the eggs one at a time, beating each one in well.

Sift together the flour and baking powder, and fold into the butter mixture. Pour into the loaf tin and bake for just over an hour, until a skewer inserted in the cake comes away clean. Leave to cool on a wire rack.

Gooey Date Loaf

110g raisins

225g stoned dates, chopped

175g sultanas

110g currants

275g butter

275ml water

400g tin condensed milk

150g plain flour

150g wholewheat flour

¾ teaspoon bicarbonate of soda

2 tablespoons marmalade

Preheat the oven to 170°C/Gas Mark 3. Grease a 20cm square cake tin, and line it with greaseproof paper.

Place the raisins, dates, sultanas and currants in a saucepan. Add the butter, water and condensed milk and bring to the boil. Turn down the heat and leave to simmer for 3 minutes, stirring now and then. Leave to cool for about 30 minutes.

Meanwhile, sift the plain flour, wholewheat flour and bicarbonate of soda into a bowl. Stir it into the cooled fruit mixture, and add the marmalade. Pour the mixture into the prepared tin and cover with a square of greaseproof paper, into the centre of which you have cut a hole about 3cm in diameter. Bake for about 2½ hours. When cooked, leave to cool on a wire rack before cutting into pieces. This will keep for a couple of weeks.

Runny Honey Cake

75g runny honey

225g plain flour

1 teaspoon ground ginger

1 teaspoon ground cinnamon

¼ teaspoon ground cloves

75g caster sugar

grated zest of 1 orange

grated zest of 1 lemon

110g cold butter

1 egg, beaten

1 teaspoon bicarbonate of soda

50g glacé cherries, chopped

Preheat the oven to 170°C/Gas Mark 3. Lightly grease a 20cm cake tin.

Warm the honey slightly in a bowl placed in hot water. Sift the flour, ginger, cinnamon and cloves into a bowl, add the sugar, orange zest and lemon zest, then rub in the cold butter until it resembles breadcrumbs. Mix in the egg, and then the warm honey. Mix the bicarbonate of soda with a little water, then add to the cake mixture. Finally add the cherries and mix well till all is combined. Pour the mixture into the cake tin and bake for about 45 minutes until springy. Leave to cool on a wire rack.

Lemon Cake

3 eggs
175g soft butter
175g caster sugar
175g self-raising flour
¼ teaspoon freshly grated nutmeg
grated zest of 4 lemons
juice of 2 lemons

Preheat the oven to 180°C/Gas Mark 4. Grease and line a 20cm cake tin.

Place all the ingredients in a bowl and beat well for a few minutes until the mixture is light and fluffy. Pour it into a tin and bake for about 1 hour until golden. Serve warm with cream, or cold.

Apple Cake

225g Bramley apples, peeled, cored and chopped
juice of 1 lemon
225g plain flour
1½ teaspoons baking powder
115g cold butter, cut into cubes
165g demerara sugar
1 egg, beaten
a little milk
½ teaspoon ground cinnamon

Preheat the oven to 180°C/Gas Mark 4. Grease and line a 20cm cake tin.

Sprinkle the lemon juice over the apple to stop it going brown. Sift together the flour and the baking powder, then rub in the butter until it resembles breadcrumbs. Stir in two-thirds of the sugar, then mix in the apple and egg and enough milk to give a soft consistency. Pour the mixture into the tin. Sprinkle over the remaining sugar and the cinnamon and bake for about 50 minutes until golden. Leave to cool on a wire rack.

Scones

MAKES ABOUT 10

225g plain flour
1 tablespoon baking powder
4 tablespoons cold butter, diced
1 egg, beaten
75ml milk
beaten egg to glaze

Preheat the oven to 220°C/Gas Mark 7. Lightly grease a baking tray.

Sift together the flour and baking powder, then rub in the diced butter until it looks like breadcrumbs. Add the egg and milk, and mix with a palette knife until you have a soft dough. Roll out to a thickness of about 2cm, then cut out the scones using a circular cutter. Place on a baking sheet and glaze with beaten egg. Bake for 7–8 minutes until golden. Cool slightly on a wire rack before serving with butter.

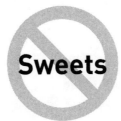

Sweets

Sweets fall into much the same category as biscuits and cakes for the nut-allergy sufferer. It's so difficult to be sure that you are avoiding nuts when all the different chocolates in a box are made in the same factory. Chocolate and nuts is such a common food combination, too. Experiment with the recipes in this section and make your own sweets at home. It's much easier than you might imagine.

Chocolate Fudge

900g sugar

275ml milk

110g butter

3 tablespoons very good-quality organic cocoa powder

juice and grated zest of 1 orange

a few drops vanilla extract

Place the sugar and milk in a large saucepan and soak for an hour. Slowly bring to the boil with all the other ingredients except the vanilla. Once it has reached boiling point, boil fast for 10–15 minutes. Do not stir any more than is necessary to keep the mixture from burning. Remove it from the heat when it begins to crystallise on the side of the saucepan. Leave for two minutes, then add the vanilla and beat well with a wooden spoon. Pour it on to a well-buttered tin and allow to cool. Score it into pieces when still slightly warm.

Home-made Toffee

350g demerara sugar

225g butter

200g golden syrup

juice and grated rind of ½ lemon

Boil all the ingredients together until, when you drop a little into a glass of cold water, it sets immediately. Pour the mixture into a greased tin. When almost set, score with a knife and loosen slightly from the tin. When quite cold, break into pieces.

Turkish Delight

700g sugar
juice and grated zest of 1 lemon
juice and grated zest of 1 orange
150ml water, plus a little extra
75g cornflour
25g gelatine
icing sugar

You will need a sugar thermometer to make this recipe. Soften the gelatine in a little water. Place the sugar, zest, juice and 150ml water in a large saucepan and bring slowly to the boil. The sugar must dissolve before it hits boiling point. Boil until the mixture reaches 110°C. Mix the cornflour with a little water and add to the syrup. Add the softened gelatine to the pan and boil until it has dissolved, stirring occasionally. Strain the liquid into tins about 3cm deep, and leave overnight to cool. Cut into cubes and dust with icing sugar.

Peppermint Creams

450g icing sugar
1 egg white
60ml double cream
peppermint essence

Mix together the icing sugar, egg white and cream. Add a few drops of peppermint essence and mix well. On a board dusted with icing sugar, roll the paste into a long sausage, then cut into slices. Leave to dry for 12 hours on a wire rack.

Chocolate Truffles

450g very good-quality cooking chocolate
275ml double cream
good organic cocoa powder for dusting

Break up the chocolate into very small, evenly sized pieces.
Bring the cream to the boil, and pour over the chocolate. Stir
until the chocolate is melted – you might need to put the bowl
over a pan of simmering water, but take care not to overheat
it. Place the bowl in the fridge for an hour or so. Then, using
a teaspoon, scoop out and fashion balls of the chocolate
mixture and dust them with cocoa powder.

Treacle Toffee

450g demerara sugar

225g black treacle

110g unsalted butter

2 tablespoons water

1 tablespoon white wine vinegar

You will need a sugar thermometer for this recipe. Lightly grease a 20cm square cake tin. Place the butter, water and vinegar into a large saucepan. Heat very gently until the butter has melted. Add the sugar and black treacle and heat very gently until the mixture has dissolved. Boil the mixture to 140°C. Remove from the heat and allow to cool slightly. Pour the mixture into the cake tin. When almost set, score with a knife and loosen slightly from the tin. When quite cold, break into pieces.

Honeycomb

225g sugar

300ml cold water

1 tablespoon golden syrup

1 teaspoon warm water

½ teaspoon bicarbonate of soda

½ teaspoon cream of tartar

For this recipe you will need a sugar thermometer. Place the sugar, water, golden syrup and cream of tartar into a large saucepan. Heat very gently until the sugar has completely dissolved. Bring to the boil and heat, without stirring, to a temperature of 155°C. Remove from the heat. Mix the bicarbonate of soda with the warm water and add to the sugar mixture, stirring gently.

Pour the mixture into a 20x30cm non-stick baking tray to a depth of about 3cm. Allow to cool for a few minutes before cutting into bite-sized squares.

Apricot Surprises

Note: Some almond-allergy sufferers may have an intolerance to apricots. Only use this recipe if you are sure it is safe.

450g sugar
300ml water
150g dried apricots
150ml warm water
50g gelatine
2 teaspoons lemon juice
caster sugar for dusting

Soak the apricots for 12 hours.

Place the apricots and water in a saucepan and cook until soft. Liquidise. You will need about 275ml purée. Place the purée in the saucepan, add the sugar and heat gently until the sugar is fully dissolved.

Place the gelatine and warm water in a bowl over a saucepan of hot water. Stir until the gelatine is fully dissolved, then stir it into the apricot mixture. Strain the mixture into a 20cm baking tray. Place in the fridge and leave to set overnight. When set, cut into squares and dust with caster sugar.

Apple Pastilles

600ml stewed apple purée

40g gelatine

75ml water

350g caster sugar

1 tablespoon lemon juice

2 teaspoons cornflour

2 teaspoons caster sugar

Place the apple purée into a small saucepan and heat through. Dissolve the gelatine in the water and add to the apple mixture. Remove from the heat, add the lemon juice and mix well. Pour the mixture into a 20x30cm non-stick baking tray to a depth of at least 3cm. Place in the fridge and leave to set overnight. Sieve together the cornflour and caster sugar. Cut the pastilles into cubes and dust with the sugar mixture.

Humbugs

450g demerara sugar
150ml water
peppermint essence

For this recipe you will need a sugar thermometer. Place the
demerara sugar into a large saucepan and heat gently until
the sugar has completely dissolved, but do not stir. Boil to a
temperature of 155°C, then add a few drops of peppermint
essence. Pour the mixture thinly on to a baking tray, leave to
cool, then cut into pieces using a pair of scissors. Wrap in
cling film to store.

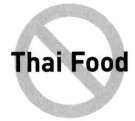

Thai Food

This is the first of three chapters which deal with the difficulty to the nut-allergy sufferer of certain ethnic cuisines. Restaurants specialising in Thai food are extremely popular, but they can pose great difficulty if you are allergic to nuts. All sorts of nuts are used regularly in Thai kitchens, so you will probably have been advised to avoid Thai restaurants altogether. But that doesn't mean you can't enjoy the food. Here are ten recipes that you can easily make at home. Enjoy!

Thai Green Curry

Note: This recipe contains coconut milk. Generally speaking, nut-allergy sufferers do not react to coconut, but some do. If you are at all unsure, try one of the other recipes. Don't take the risk.

SERVES 4

750g lean chicken breast, chopped
3 tablespoons sunflower oil
4 large flat mushrooms
400ml coconut milk
400ml stock
2 tablespoons coriander leaves

For the Thai paste:
4 stalks lemon grass, outer leaves removed, chopped
4 small green chillies (or more if you think you can handle it!),
   seeded and chopped
1 small onion, peeled and chopped
4 fat garlic cloves, peeled and chopped
4 cm piece ginger, peeled and chopped
4 tablespoons coriander leaves, chopped
juice and zest of 1 lime
1 tablespoon fish sauce
lots of freshly ground black pepper

Place all the Thai paste ingredients in a food processor and blitz until you have a bright green paste.

Fry the chicken in the sunflower oil until it is just cooked, then add the mushrooms and the Thai paste. Cook for a minute, then add the coconut milk and stock. Bring to the boil and leave to simmer gently for about 10 minutes. Scatter the coriander leaves over the top, and serve with boiled rice.

Vermicelli Soup

SERVES 4

1 litre chicken stock

1 onion, chopped

2 stalks lemon grass, outer leaves removed, chopped

3 kaffir lime leaves, shredded

juice of 1 lime

2 garlic cloves, chopped

2 small red chillies, seeded and chopped

4cm piece ginger, peeled and finely chopped

2 tablespoons fish sauce

2 teaspoons demerara sugar

120g vermicelli noodles, soaked in water according to the
    packet instructions and drained

2 tablespoons coriander leaves, roughly chopped

Place the stock, onion, lemon grass, lime leaves, lime juice,
garlic, chillies and ginger in a saucepan. Bring to the boil and
simmer for 20 minutes. Stir in the fish sauce and sugar. Allow
the sugar to dissolve, add the noodles and cook for 1 minute.
Add the coriander and serve.

Chicken and Mushroom Soup

SERVES 4

2 garlic cloves, finely chopped

1 tablespoon coriander leaves and stalks

1 teaspoon freshly ground black pepper

1 tablespoon sunflower oil

1 litre chicken stock

handful of dried mushrooms, soaked in boiling water according
to the packet instructions and roughly chopped

1 tablespoon fish sauce

120g lean chicken breast, cut into bite-sized pieces

50g spring onions, finely chopped

Use a pestle and mortar to pound the garlic, coriander and pepper to a paste. In a large saucepan or wok, heat the oil. Add the paste and cook for a couple of minutes. Add the stock, mushrooms and fish sauce. Bring to the boil, then simmer for 5 minutes. Slide the chicken into the soup, and simmer very gently for another 5 minutes. Add the spring onions and serve.

Spiced Pork and Prawn Toasts

SERVES 4

175g minced pork

50g cooked peeled prawns, finely chopped

1 garlic clove, finely chopped

2 spring onions, finely chopped

1 tablespoon coriander leaves, chopped

2 large eggs, beaten

2 teaspoons fish sauce

4 slices stale bread

sunflower oil for frying

freshly ground black pepper

Mix together the first five ingredients with half the beaten egg. Spread the mixture well over the slices of bread, then brush with the remaining egg. Cut off the crusts, then divide each slice into four squares.

Heat the oil to 190°C in a deep-fat fryer. Fry the toasts a few at a time for about 4 minutes. They should be good and crisp. They will need turning over halfway through, and you will probably find it easier to start them off pork-side down. Keep them warm in the oven until they are all cooked, then serve immediately.

Thai Garlic Prawns

SERVES 4

2 tablespoons sunflower oil

4 cloves garlic, chopped

1cm piece ginger, peeled and finely chopped

16 large raw prawns

2 tablespoons fish sauce

2 tablespoons coriander leaves, chopped

freshly ground pepper

lettuce leaves to serve

Heat the oil in a wok, then add the garlic. Stir-fry for 2 minutes. Add the ginger, fry for 1 minute, then add the prawns and stir-fry for 3 minutes, or until they start to become opaque. Add the fish sauce and lots of black pepper. Cook for 2 minutes, then serve on a bed of lettuce.

Coriander-roasted Chicken

SERVES 4

handful of coriander leaves
½ tablespoon freshly ground black pepper
3 garlic cloves, chopped
juice of 1 lime
3 teaspoons fish sauce
4 large chicken pieces, bone in

In a food processor, mix together the first five ingredients. Slash the skin of the chicken pieces, and smear the mixture over the chicken. Cover and leave in the fridge for 3 hours.

Preheat the grill. Grill the chicken for about 10 minutes, or until it is golden and cooked through. Serve with rice.

Thai-style Mussels

SERVES 2

700g mussels, cleaned, de-bearded and rinsed
6cm piece ginger, quartered
3 stalks lemon grass, outer leaves discarded, chopped

For the dipping sauce:
1 large garlic clove, finely chopped
2 small red chillies, seeded and finely chopped
juice of 1 lemon
1 tablespoon light soy sauce
2 tablespoons fish sauce
1 teaspoon sugar

Discard any mussels that are open. Place the mussels, ginger and lemon grass in a large saucepan, and add about 1cm of water. Cover and place on a medium heat for 10–15 minutes. If there are any mussels that have not now opened, discard them.

Combine all the dipping sauce ingredients together, and serve with the hot mussels.

Fried Noodles Thai-style

SERVES 4

3 tablespoons sunflower oil
3 garlic cloves, finely chopped
1 tablespoon fish sauce
juice of 2 limes
2 large eggs, beaten
350g vermicelli, soaked according to the instructions
   on the packet
150g cooked peeled prawns
150g bean sprouts
4 spring onions, finely sliced
slices of lime and coriander leaves to garnish

Heat the oil in a wok, add the garlic and stir-fry until golden. Add the fish sauce, lime juice and eggs. Stir quickly for a few seconds, then add the noodles. Stir well so that the noodles are well coated, then add the bean sprouts and the spring onions. When it is all hot, serve garnished with slices of lime and coriander leaves.

Lemony Lemon Sole

SERVES 1–2

1 lemon sole (or you could use plaice)
4 tablespoons sunflower oil
2 garlic cloves, finely chopped
3 small red chillies, finely chopped
2 tablespoons fish sauce
4 tablespoons water
juice of 2 lemons
2 tablespoons sugar
2 tablespoons flour

Fry the sole in 2 tablespoons of sunflower oil and put to one side. Heat the remaining oil and fry the garlic until just golden. Add the chillies, fry for 30 seconds, then add the liquids and the sugar. Bring to the boil. Mix the flour with 2 tablespoons of water and add to the sauce, a teaspoon at a time, so that it thickens. You may not need to use all the flour mixture. Pour the sauce over the fish and serve.

Pork and Mange Tout Stir-fry

SERVES 4

3 tablespoons sunflower oil
2 garlic cloves, finely chopped
130g minced pork
500g mange tout
1 tablespoon fish sauce
60g cooked peeled prawns, finely chopped
freshly ground black pepper

Heat the oil in a wok, then add the garlic and stir-fry until just golden. Add the pork, and stir-fry for 3 minutes. Add the mange tout and stir-fry until just cooked – about 3 minutes. Stir in the remaining ingredients, stir-fry for 1 minute, then serve.

Chinese Food

The next ethnic cuisine which the nut-allergy sufferer needs to be very careful of is Chinese. Nuts abound in Chinese cooking and, as with Thai food, nut-allergy sufferers are rightly advised to avoid Chinese restaurants. But that doesn't mean to say that you can't enjoy your own nut-free Chinese food at home. All the recipes in this chapter are quite simple to prepare, so why not have a go?

Sweet and Sour Pork

SERVES 4

3 tablespoons sunflower oil
1 small onion, peeled and finely chopped
100g red pepper, seeded and finely diced
100g green pepper, seeded and finely diced
1 large garlic clove, finely chopped
2cm piece ginger, peeled and finely chopped
1 tablespoon dark soy sauce
1 tablespoon white wine vinegar
2 teaspoons rice vinegar
1 tablespoon tomato purée
50ml unsweetened pineapple juice
20g runny honey
150g fresh or tinned pineapple, diced
2 tablespoons cornflour
1 tablespoon chilli sauce
1 egg, beaten
500g lean pork, cut into bite-sized cubes
salt and freshly ground black pepper

Heat 1 tablespoon of sunflower oil in a pan. Add the onion, peppers, garlic and ginger and fry until just soft. Add the soy sauce, vinegars, tomato purée, pineapple juice and honey and bring to the boil. Add the diced pineapple and simmer very gently for about 10 minutes. Dilute 1 tablespoon of cornflour in a little water, then add to the sauce. Season, and simmer for a few more minutes.

Mix together the remaining cornflour and the beaten egg, then heat the remaining sunflower oil. Dunk the pork in the cornflour mixture and fry on a fairly high heat for about 5 minutes until cooked. Add the pork to the sauce, and heat through. Serve with rice.

Barbecue Spare Ribs

SERVES 4

1kg spare ribs

1 tablespoon balsamic vinegar

2 tablespoons tomato ketchup

3 tablespoons runny honey

2 tablespoons soy sauce

2 tablespoons red wine vinegar

1 level teaspoon English mustard powder

65ml water

½ teaspoon paprika

salt and freshly ground black pepper

Put the ribs in a large saucepan of salted water, bring to the boil and simmer for 15 minutes. Place the remaining ingredients in a saucepan, bring to the boil and simmer for 5 minutes, stirring occasionally. Strain the ribs in a colander, put them in a bowl, then pour over the barbecue sauce. Turn frequently until cool.

You are now ready to cook the ribs, which can be done on the barbecue or under a hot grill. Either way, they will take about 10 minutes, and you will need to keep brushing them with the barbecue sauce.

Barbecue-style Pork

SERVES 4

4cm piece ginger, peeled and grated

1 large onion, peeled and very finely chopped

2 garlic cloves, peeled and very finely chopped

90ml light soy sauce

70ml sherry

1 large pork fillet, about 750g

2 tablespoons runny honey

1 tablespoon dark soy sauce

1 tablespoon rice wine

1 tablespoon sunflower oil

salt and freshly ground black pepper

Mix together the ginger, onion, garlic, light soy sauce and sherry. Halve the fillet lengthways and marinate overnight in the mixture.

Preheat the oven to 200°C/Gas Mark 6. Mix together the remaining ingredients, which you will use to baste the pork. Remove the pork from the marinade and place on a wire rack on a baking tray. Pour a little water into the bottom of the baking tray, brush with the basting liquid and roast for 15 minutes. Turn the fillet over, baste again, reduce the heat to 180°C/Gas Mark 4, and cook for another 20 minutes, basting every 5 minutes. Remove from the oven, baste a final time and leave for 5 minutes. Slice very thinly and serve.

Chicken in Rice Wine

SERVES 4

1 chicken
4 spring onions, roughly chopped
6cm piece ginger, roughly chopped
1 teaspoon peppercorns
1 teaspoon salt
2 tablespoons dark soy sauce
1 tablespoon demerara sugar
100ml rice wine

Place the chicken in a large pan. Add the spring onions, ginger, peppercorns and salt. Cover with water, bring to the boil, then simmer for 45 minutes until the chicken is cooked. Leave to cool in the water, then remove it, cut it up and place the pieces of chicken in a shallow dish. Place the remaining ingredients in a saucepan and heat until the sugar is dissolved. Pour over the chicken, leave to cool and serve.

Duck and Mange Tout Stir-fry

SERVES 4

2 tablespoons soy sauce

1 tablespoon rice wine

1 teaspoon sugar

4 duck breasts, thinly sliced

2 tablespoons sunflower oil

1 onion, finely chopped

2 garlic cloves, finely chopped

6cm piece ginger, peeled and finely chopped

3 small green chillies, seeded and finely chopped

400g mange tout

salt and freshly ground pepper

Mix together the soy sauce, rice wine and sugar. Add the duck breasts and marinate for about 1 hour. Heat the oil in a large wok, then add the onion, garlic, ginger and chillies. Stir-fry for 1 minute before adding the duck slices. Stir-fry for 5 minutes, then remove the duck from the pan. Add the mange tout, stir-fry for two minutes, then return the duck to the pan. Serve with rice.

Peking Duck

SERVES 4

1 large duck
1 tablespoon runny honey
1 teaspoon salt
1 teaspoon five-spice powder
250ml warm water

Place the duck in a pan, and cover with boiling water. Remove from the pan and dry thoroughly. It is important that the duck is very dry. The traditional Chinese method is to hang the duck in a dry place overnight and let it drip-dry – you could try that!

Mix together the remaining ingredients and allow to dry thoroughly. Preheat the oven to 200°C/Gas Mark 6. Place the duck on a rack in a baking tray, pour an inch of water into the tray, and roast for about 1½ hours, or until cooked. Baste with the sauce every 15 minutes.

When the duck is cooked, allow it to rest for 20 minutes, then carve and shred the meat. Serve with pancakes and shredded spring onions and cucumber. (The pancakes can be pre-bought from the supermarket – but do check that they have not been made with sesame oil.)

Chinese Steamed Fish

SERVES 4

1 large sea bass, cleaned
sea salt
juice of ½ lemon
1 tablespoon soy sauce
6 spring onions, finely chopped
4 garlic cloves, finely chopped
2cm piece ginger, peeled and finely chopped
2 tablespoons sunflower oil

For this recipe you will need a fish steamer. Slash the fish a few times on each side, then rub a little salt all over the fish. Mix together the lemon and soy sauce, and rub this into the flesh. Rub half the spring onions, garlic cloves and ginger into the flesh, then place in the steamer over bubbling water and steam for about 10 minutes until cooked. Quickly fry the remaining spring onions, garlic and ginger in the sunflower oil, spoon over the fish and serve.

Chinese-style Scallops

SERVES 4

1 small red chilli, seeded and finely sliced
2cm piece ginger, peeled and finely chopped
1 garlic clove, finely chopped
4 tablespoons dark soy sauce
12 fresh scallops, cleaned but still in their shells
coriander leaves to garnish

Mix together the chilli, ginger, garlic and soy sauce. Spoon a little over each scallop. Steam the scallops for about 1 minute over a pan of boiling water. Remove, add a little more of the sauce, garnish with coriander leaves and serve immediately.

Chow Mein

SERVES 4

4 tablespoons sunflower oil

12 large prawns, peeled and de-veined

1 skinless chicken breast, thinly sliced

200g bean sprouts

350g egg noodles, cooked in hot water according to the
    packet instructions

2 tablespoons light soy sauce

3 spring onions, sliced

2 small red chillies, seeded and finely sliced

salt and freshly ground black pepper

Heat half the oil in a wok. Add the prawns and chicken, and stir-fry for about 5 minutes until cooked. Set aside and keep warm. Heat the remaining oil, add the bean sprouts and stir-fry for 2 minutes. Add the noodles, prawns, chicken and soy sauce, season and stir-fry for 1 minute. Serve garnished with the spring onions and chillies.

Fried Rice

SERVES 4

3 tablespoons sunflower oil

2 small onions, finely chopped

white basmati rice measured up to the 225ml level in
  a measuring jug

450ml boiling water

1 teaspoon salt

3 rashers streaky bacon, finely chopped

75g defrosted frozen peas

2 large eggs, beaten

1 tablespoon soy sauce

Heat 1 tablespoon of oil in a large saucepan. Add half the onion and fry for 2 minutes until they start to brown. Add the rice, and stir till it is completely coated with oil. Pour in the boiling water, stir, cover and simmer on the lowest heat for 15 minutes. When cooked, transfer to a bowl and leave to cool.

In a wok, heat the remaining oil, then add the bacon and the rest of the onion. Stir-fry until the bacon is crispy. Next, add the peas and stir-fry for 30 seconds, then add the rice and stir-fry for 30 seconds. Now add the beaten egg and stir-fry until it is cooked. Sprinkle over the soy sauce and serve.

Indian Food

This is the final chapter on ethnic cuisines that are difficult for the nut-allergy sufferer. Like Thai and Chinese, Indian food relies heavily on the use of nuts. It's fantastically popular, though, and one of the most difficult foods for nut-allergy sufferers to avoid. But, even though your local Indian restaurant might be out of bounds, it doesn't mean you can't enjoy some great Indian food. Simply use these recipes to satisfy that craving for a curry.

Indian Baked Chicken

SERVES 4–6

1 tablespoon ground cumin

1 teaspoon hot chilli powder (or mild if you prefer
   things a little less fiery)

1 tablespoon ground turmeric

1 tablespoon paprika

1 teaspoon freshly ground black pepper

2 teaspoons salt

3 garlic cloves, very finely chopped

juice of 3 lemons

8 chicken pieces on the bone

3 tablespoons sunflower oil

Mix the first eight ingredients in a bowl, then smear the mixture well all over the chicken pieces. Leave to marinate in the fridge for 2–3 hours.

Preheat the oven to 200°C/Gas Mark 6. Brush the chicken pieces with sunflower oil, then bake for about 50 minutes, or until cooked. Skim the fat off any juices in the pan, then pour the juices into a saucepan. Boil vigorously until reduced by half, pour over the chicken and serve with rice.

Indian-style Kebabs

SERVES 4

700g lean lamb, cut into cubes

3 tablespoons olive oil

8 cherry tomatoes, cut in half

1 large onion, quartered and split into pieces

1 small yellow pepper, seeded and cut into pieces

2 teaspoons mild curry powder

1 teaspoon ground cumin

1 teaspoon ground coriander

juice of 1 lemon

200g natural yoghurt

salt and freshly ground black pepper

Season the lamb with salt and pepper and marinate in the olive oil for 2 hours, turning every ½ hour. Add the tomatoes, onions and yellow pepper. Mix together the spices, lemon juice and yoghurt, then add to the meat and vegetables. Mix well, and leave for another 2 hours.

Take 4 long skewers, and thread the lamb and vegetables along them, making sure that everything is nicely mixed up. Grill for about 15 minutes under a hot grill, turning them every 2 minutes and basting them with the remaining marinade. Serve with rice.

Indian Fried Cauliflower

SERVES 4

2 teaspoons coriander seeds

1 teaspoon turmeric

4 tablespoons olive oil

1 large cauliflower, broken into florets

1 onion, finely chopped

20g butter

1 large garlic clove, finely chopped

salt and freshly ground black pepper

Crush the coriander seeds with the turmeric, using a pestle and mortar. Heat the oil in a wok until it is bubbling hot, then add the cauliflower. Stir-fry for 2 minutes, then add the coriander, turmeric and onion. Stir-fry for a further 5 minutes, then season with salt and pepper. Add the butter and garlic, cook for 1 more minute, and serve immediately.

Spicy Lemon Chicken with Herbs

SERVES 4–6

5cm piece ginger, peeled and roughly chopped

4 tablespoons sunflower oil

8 chicken pieces on the bone

6 garlic cloves, peeled and finely chopped

150g fresh coriander leaves, finely chopped

1 small green chilli, seeded and finely chopped

¼ teaspoon cayenne pepper

2 teaspoons ground cumin

1 teaspoon ground coriander

½ teaspoon ground turmeric

juice of 2 lemons

salt and freshly ground black pepper

Place the ginger in a food processor and blitz with 5 tablespoons of water till you have a thin paste. Heat the oil in a large saucepan and fry the chicken, in two batches, until it is golden brown all over. Remove the chicken, add the garlic and fry until just golden. Reduce the heat and add the ginger paste. Stir-fry for 2 minutes. Add the coriander, chilli, cayenne pepper, ground cumin, ground coriander and turmeric. Season with salt and pepper, then stir-fry for 1 minute. Return the chicken to the pan, adding 100ml water and the lemon juice. Cover and cook for 45 minutes or until the chicken is cooked through. Serve with rice.

Prawn Curry

SERVES 4

1 large onion, peeled and chopped

6 garlic cloves

3cm piece ginger, peeled and chopped

4 tablespoons sunflower oil

3cm piece cinnamon stick

5 cardamom pods

3 bay leaves

2 teaspoons ground cumin

1 teaspoon ground coriander

4 tomatoes, peeled and finely chopped

5 tablespoons natural yoghurt

½ teaspoon ground turmeric

¼ teaspoon cayenne pepper

good pinch of salt

400g raw prawns, peeled and deveined

good handful of coriander leaves, chopped

Put the onion, garlic and ginger in a food processor. Add 3 tablespoons of water and blend to a paste. Heat the oil in a large saucepan, then add the cinnamon stick, cardamom pods and bay leaves. Stir, then add the onion paste. Stir-fry for about 5 minutes until golden brown, then add the ground cumin and ground coriander. Stir-fry for 2 minutes, then add the yoghurt gradually, stirring bit by bit so that it incorporates itself well. Add the turmeric and cayenne pepper, then add 300ml water. Mix well, and add the salt and the prawns. Bring to the boil, then cook for about 5 minutes, or until the prawns are just cooked through. Serve with rice and garnish with the fresh coriander.

Spicy Baked Cod

SERVES 4

4 thick cod steaks
1 teaspoon salt
½ teaspoon hot chilli powder
½ teaspoon ground turmeric
sunflower oil for frying
1 teaspoon fennel seeds
2 teaspoons black mustard seeds
1 large onion, peeled and finely chopped
1 garlic clove, peeled and finely chopped
2 teaspoons ground cumin
400g tin chopped tomatoes

Preheat the oven to 180°C/Gas Mark 4. Rub the cod steaks with half the salt, half the chilli powder and the turmeric. Heat about 4 tablespoons of sunflower oil in a large saucepan. Add the fennel and mustard seeds, stir, then add the onions and garlic. Stir-fry until the onions begin to turn brown. Add the cumin, remaining salt and remaining cayenne. Stir, then add the tomatoes. Bring to the boil, cover and simmer for 20 minutes.

Heat another 4 tablespoons of oil in a large saucepan. Fry the cod steaks until just brown on both sides. Place in a baking dish, then pour over the tomato sauce. Put in the oven and cook for about 20 minutes or until the fish is done.

Devilled Mackerel

SERVES 4

4 large mackerel, filleted
bunch of fresh coriander, finely chopped
2 small red chillies, seeded and finely chopped
juice of 1 lemon
salt and freshly ground black pepper

Slash the mackerel skin on both sides with a sharp knife. Mix together the coriander, chilli, lemon juice and plenty of seasoning, and rub this marinade all over the fish. Leave for 1 hour, then grill for 4 minutes each side.

Spicy Vegetables

SERVES 4–6

6 garlic cloves
5cm piece ginger, peeled and chopped
5 tablespoons sunflower oil
2 teaspoons cumin seeds
½ teaspoon dried chilli
2 teaspoons ground coriander
225g tomatoes, peeled and finely chopped
250g green beans, chopped into 2cm pieces
250g cauliflower, cut into small florets
250g carrot, cut into very thin batons
juice of 1 large lemon
salt and freshly ground black pepper

Place the garlic and ginger in a food processor. Add 100ml water and blend till you have a smooth paste. Heat a large saucepan, and add the sunflower oil. Add the cumin seeds and crushed chilli and, as soon as they start to change colour, add the garlic mixture. Stir-fry for 1 minute before adding the coriander and the tomatoes. Stir-fry for 2 minutes. Add the vegetables and season well. Add 250ml water and bring to the boil. Simmer, covered, for about 10 minutes or until the vegetables are tender. Add the lemon juice, then boil furiously, uncovered, until the liquid has evaporated, and serve.

Vegetable Bhaji

SERVES 4–6

3 tablespoons sunflower oil

1½ teaspoons cumin seeds

1 teaspoon dried chilli

150g onion, roughly chopped

150g carrots, diced

150g cooked frozen peas

150g cooked potatoes, diced

salt and sugar to season

2 spring onions

Heat the oil in a large frying pan. Add the cumin seeds, chilli and onion and stir-fry for about 5 minutes. Add the carrots and peas, and stir-fry for about 1 minute. Turn down the heat, then cover and cook for a few minutes until the carrots are tender. Add the potatoes and season with sugar and salt. Turn up the heat and cook for another 3 minutes. Mix in the spring onions and serve.

Indian Potato Stew

SERVES 4–6

275g cooked peeled potatoes

400g button mushrooms

3cm piece ginger, peeled

5 garlic cloves

4 tablespoons sunflower oil

½ teaspoon ground turmeric

1 teaspoon cumin seeds

3 cardamom pods

4 large tomatoes, peeled and finely chopped

1 teaspoon ground cumin

½ teaspoon ground coriander

½ teaspoon hot chilli powder

salt

Cut the potatoes into 2cm cubes. Wipe the mushrooms with a piece of kitchen towel. Blitz the ginger and garlic in a food processor with 3 tbsp water until you have a smooth purée. Season the potatoes with salt, then sprinkle half the turmeric over them and mix well. Heat the oil in a large saucepan, add the potatoes and stir-fry until golden brown. Remove the potatoes and add the cumin seeds and cardamom pods to the pan. Add the tomatoes, garlic paste, cumin and coriander and stir-fry to a thick sauce. Add the remaining turmeric and the chilli powder, then pour in 250ml water, the potatoes and the mushrooms. Season well with salt. Bring to the boil, cover and simmer for 5 minutes. Remove the cardamom pods and serve.

Vegetarian Food

Nuts are one of the most common fallbacks for the vegetarian. The ubiquitous nut roast, of course, is a very common Sunday lunch alternative; but nuts crop up elsewhere in vegetarian cookery all the time. This can make life very difficult for the vegetarian nut-allergy sufferer, although it doesn't mean you can't eat well. This chapter contains some very good nut-free vegetarian recipes that can be served as main courses. And remember – you don't have to be a vegetarian to enjoy them …

Gratin of Courgettes

SERVES 4

3 tablespoons olive oil

8 large courgettes, sliced

2 large garlic cloves, finely chopped

1 medium onion, sliced

250g Cheddar cheese, thinly sliced

8 large tomatoes, peeled and sliced

8 tablespoons Parmesan cheese, grated

1 teaspoon dried thyme

salt and freshly ground black pepper

Preheat the oven to 190°C/Gas Mark 5. Heat the oil in a large frying pan and fry the courgettes and garlic in batches (do not overcrowd the pan) until golden. In a deep baking dish, arrange alternate layers of courgette, Cheddar and tomato. Finish with a layer of grated Parmesan, sprinkle with the dried thyme, and season well with salt and pepper. Bake for 30 minutes and serve with salad.

Vegetable Casserole

SERVES 4

2 tablespoons sunflower oil

10 shallots, peeled and left whole

1 tablespoon wholemeal flour

2 tablespoons paprika

pinch of cayenne pepper

400g tin tomatoes

275ml hot water

½ medium cauliflower, cut into sprigs

225g carrots, roughly chopped

225g courgettes, roughly chopped

300g new potatoes, halved

½ red pepper, seeded and chopped

200ml yoghurt

salt and freshly ground black pepper

Preheat the oven to 180°C/Gas Mark 4. Heat the oil in a large saucepan and fry the shallots until they start to soften. Stir in the flour, 1½ tablespoons paprika and the cayenne pepper. Cook for 1–2 minutes, stirring occasionally, then add the tomatoes and the water. Bring to the boil, stirring constantly, then add the cauliflower, carrots, courgettes and potatoes. Season with salt and pepper, then transfer everything to a casserole dish. Cover and bake for 45 minutes. Stir in the yoghurt, and sprinkle with the remaining paprika. Serve with rice.

Piperade

SERVES 4

100g butter
1 small onion, finely chopped
3 garlic cloves, finely chopped
4 red peppers, seeded, sliced and blanched for 1 minute in
boiling water
450g tomatoes, skinned, seeded and chopped
8 eggs
4 tablespoons milk

Melt the butter in a large frying pan and add the onion and garlic. When they begin to change colour, add the peppers. Cook for 5 minutes, then add the tomatoes. Season well and allow to simmer gently for 10 minutes. Beat the eggs, add the milk and season. Pour the eggs into the pan and cook for 4 minutes until the eggs are set. Serve with bread and butter, and a green salad.

Provençale Stuffed Tomatoes

SERVES 4

8 large tomatoes
2 tablespoons olive oil
2 onions, finely chopped
2 garlic cloves, finely chopped
8 tablespoons fresh breadcrumbs
4 anchovies, rinsed and mashed
a little butter
salt and freshly ground black pepper

Preheat the oven to 190°C/Gas Mark 5. Cut the tomatoes in half widthways and scoop the insides out into a bowl. Place the halved tomatoes in a greased baking dish. Heat the oil in a frying pan, add the onions and garlic, and cook gently until soft. Strain the tomato pulp through a sieve, then add the juice to the onion and garlic mixture. Add the breadcrumbs and anchovies, and season with salt and pepper. Mix well and stuff the tomatoes with the mixture. Dot the tomatoes with butter, then bake for 30 minutes and serve.

Cheese Soufflé

SERVES 2

25g butter
15g flour
150ml milk
3 egg yolks, beaten
4 egg whites
40g Parmesan, grated
40g Cheddar, grated

Preheat the oven to 190°C/Gas Mark 5. Grease a soufflé dish. Melt the butter in a large saucepan, stir in the flour, then add the milk bit by bit. Bring to the boil, stirring constantly. Add the cheese and allow to cool slightly before mixing in the egg yolks. Whisk the egg whites until they are very stiff, then fold them into the cheese mixture. Turn into the soufflé dish, and bake for about 20 minutes until risen and golden. Serve immediately.

Vegetable Hotpot

SERVES 4

2 onions, sliced

4 carrots, sliced

1 small swede, sliced

2 parsnips, sliced

1 small celeriac, finely chopped

2 leeks, sliced

2 garlic cloves, chopped

1 tablespoon rosemary, chopped

1 tablespoon parsley, chopped

350ml vegetable stock

1½ tablespoons plain flour

700g potatoes, thinly sliced

50g butter

salt and freshly ground black pepper

Preheat the oven to 190°C/Gas Mark 5. Arrange all the vegetables except the potatoes in alternate layers in a large casserole, seasoning well with garlic, herbs, salt and pepper between each layer. Whisk the stock into the flour and pour into the pot. Arrange the potatoes on the top, then dot with the butter. Cover tightly and bake for at least 1 hour until the vegetables are tender. Place under a hot grill until the potatoes turn golden, then serve.

Spinach and Mushroom Roulade

SERVES 6–8

450g fresh spinach, washed, stalks removed

40g butter

4 eggs, separated

freshly grated nutmeg

50g Gruyère, grated

400g mushrooms, finely chopped

25g plain flour

200ml single cream

2 tablespoons chives, finely chopped

Preheat the oven to 190°C/Gas Mark 5. Line a 20x30cm Swiss roll tin with baking paper – it needs to extend to about 2cm round the side of the tin. Place the spinach in a large saucepan, cover and cook until tender. Drain well and chop finely. Place the chopped spinach in a bowl, beat in 20g butter and the egg yolks. Season with salt, pepper and nutmeg. Whisk the egg whites until stiff, then fold them into the spinach mixture. Spread the mixture into the tin, sprinkle with half the cheese, then bake for 10 minutes.

Meanwhile, melt the butter in a saucepan and sauté the mushrooms until soft. Stir in the flour, cook for 1 minute then add the cream gradually, stirring all the time. Bring to the boil, stirring constantly, then stir in the chives. Spread this over the spinach roulade, then roll it up, peeling away the baking paper. Transfer to a baking dish, sprinkle with the remaining cheese and bake for 5 minutes. Slice and serve.

Filo Spinach Pie

SERVES 6–8

1.5kg spinach leaves, washed, stalks removed

2 tablespoons olive oil

1 large onion, finely chopped

1 teaspoon dried thyme

4 eggs, beaten

500g cottage cheese

150g Gruyère, grated

12 sheets frozen filo pastry, thawed

50 butter

salt and freshly ground black pepper

Preheat the oven to 190°C/Gas Mark 5. Place the spinach in a large saucepan, cover and cook in its own moisture until tender. Drain it well, then chop it finely. Heat the oil in large saucepan, add the onion and cook until soft. Do not allow the onion to go brown. Add the spinach and oregano, then remove from the heat and allow to cool. Stir in the eggs, cottage cheese and Parmesan. Season with salt, pepper and a little nutmeg.

Melt the butter, then brush it over a 20x30cm baking dish. Cover the bottom and sides, extending about 2cm above the sides, with 6 sheets of filo pastry. Brush with butter, then spoon in the spinach mixture. Cover with the remaining filo pastry, tucking the edges neatly over the side of the mixture. Brush the top with butter and bake for about 20 minutes until golden brown. Serve hot.

Juicy Mushroom Sandwich

SERVES 1

50g soft butter
1 garlic clove, chopped
1 tablespoon fresh parsley, chopped
salt and freshly ground black pepper
1 large flat mushroom, wiped
1 soft bap (make sure it comes from a nut-free source)

Preheat oven to 190°C/Gas Mark 5. Mix together the butter, garlic, parsley, salt and pepper. Smear it over the inside of the mushroom, place on a baking tray and bake for 15–20 minutes. Serve inside the bap with all the buttery juices.

Leek and Stilton Soup

SERVES 4

400g leeks, roughly chopped
50g butter
2 potatoes, peeled and diced
1 litre water
300g Stilton, rind removed and crumbled
freshly ground black pepper
cream to serve

Melt the butter in a saucepan, add the leeks, cover and leave to sweat for about 15 minutes or until soft. Do not allow them to brown. Add the potatoes and cook for a further 5 minutes. Add the water, bring to the boil, then simmer for 20 minutes until the potato is soft. Add the crumbled Stilton, then liquidise. Season with pepper and serve with a swirl of cream in the bowl.

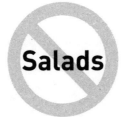

Salads

Beware the innocent salad! They so often contain walnuts, peanuts and all sorts of other nuts. The dressings can be treacherous too, sometimes being made with unrefined peanut oil. In this chapter you will find some great salads, and a selection of interesting dressings to go with them.

Caesar Salad

SERVES 4

2 thick slices white bread, crusts removed and
    cut into squares
olive oil for frying
1 egg
1 garlic clove, crushed
juice of 1 lemon
1 teaspoon Dijon mustard
150ml extra virgin olive oil
1 large crisp lettuce (iceberg or Chinese leaf
    would be suitable)
50g tin anchovy fillets
75g Parmesan cheese, thinly sliced

Heat some oil in a frying pan and, when it is hot, add the bread. Fry till golden on one side, then turn over and fry till golden on the other side. You might need to add more oil if it has all been absorbed. Remove the croutons from the pan and drain on some kitchen towel.

Whisk the egg together with the garlic, lemon juice, mustard and olive oil. Put the lettuce in a salad bowl, toss together with the dressing, anchovy fillets, Parmesan and croutons, and serve.

Provençale Tomato Salad

SERVES 4

12 large, ripe tomatoes, skinned and cut in two widthways
3 large garlic cloves, finely chopped
4 tablespoons extra virgin olive oil
2 tablespoons balsamic vinegar
handful of your favourite black olives, stones
    removed and finely chopped
handful of fresh basil leaves
salt and freshly ground black pepper

Preheat the oven to 190°C/Gas Mark 5. Place the tomatoes flesh side up in a roasting dish, sprinkle with garlic and drizzle with 2 tablespoons olive oil. Season well with salt and pepper. Roast for about 1 hour. Transfer to a serving dish, pour any pan juices over the tomatoes and leave to cool. Sprinkle with the black olives and ripped-up basil, and serve.

Avocado and Mozzarella Salad

SERVES 4

250g mozzarella cheese
2 ripe avocadoes
handful of fresh basil leaves
1 clove garlic, crushed
1 teaspoon Dijon mustard
1 tablespoon white wine vinegar
5 tablespoons extra virgin olive oil
salt and freshly ground black pepper

Slice the mozzarella into 5mm slices. Peel, stone and slice the avocados similarly. Arrange the two between four plates and scatter with ripped-up basil leaves. Make a dressing by putting the garlic, mustard, vinegar and olive oil in a jam jar with a screw-top lid and shaking vigorously. Pour over the salad and serve.

Tomato, Raisin and Herb Salad

SERVES 4

8 ripe tomatoes, peeled
3 tablespoons fresh mixed herbs (whichever you like),
    finely chopped
75g raisins, roughly chopped
1 teaspoon Dijon mustard
1 tablespoon extra virgin olive oil
juice of ½ lemon
1 teaspoon honey
salt and freshly ground black pepper

Quarter the tomatoes and mix with the raisins and herbs. Make a dressing from the mustard, oil, lemon, honey and seasoning by putting all the ingredients in a screw-top jar and shaking well. Pour over the salad and chill before serving.

Mashed Potato Salad

SERVES 4–6

750g potatoes
knob of butter
100ml hot milk
3 tablespoons cooked beetroot, finely chopped
1 small onion, finely chopped
1 garlic clove, finely chopped
a bunch of watercress and a handful of chopped chives to serve
salt and freshly ground black pepper

Peel, boil and mash the potatoes. Add the butter and hot milk, season well and beat to a smooth purée. Cover with a piece of cling film and leave until cold. Add the beetroot, onion and garlic, mix well and season again if you think it needs it. Place on a serving dish. Arrange the watercress around the potatoes and sprinkle with chives.

Pear and Watercress Salad

SERVES 4

6 tablespoons olive oil

2 tablespoons white wine vinegar

1 teaspoon English mustard

2 bunches of watercress

4 ripe pears

salt and freshly ground black pepper

First, make the dressing. Place the olive oil, vinegar, mustard and seasoning in a screw-top jar and shake well. Chop the watercress finely, and mix it with the dressing. Peel, core and slice the pears, arrange them on four plates and then top generously with the watercress dressing, making sure the pears are covered. Chill before serving.

Salade Niçoise

SERVES 4

4 small tuna steaks
1 lettuce
4 tablespoons extra virgin olive oil
2 tablespoons white wine vinegar
4 ripe tomatoes, peeled, seeded and quartered
10cm piece cucumber, peeled and cut into
    bite-sized chunks
100g new potatoes, cooked and sliced
100g French beans, cooked
2 hard-boiled eggs
1 tin anchovy fillets, drained
handful of pitted black olives

Grill the tuna steaks under a hot grill. They need to be cooked on the outside and slightly pink on the inside. Cut into slices. Arrange the lettuce in a salad bowl. Make a little dressing from the oil and vinegar, and sprinkle this over the lettuce. Now arrange the tuna, tomatoes, cucumber, potatoes, beans and hard-boiled eggs in the bowl. Arrange the anchovy fillets and olives over the top, and serve.

Creamy Green Salad

SERVES 4

2 tablespoons tarragon vinegar

2 teaspoons Dijon mustard

2 egg yolks

200ml olive oil

3 tablespoons grated pecorino cheese

bowlful of your favourite salad leaves

Place the vinegar, mustard, egg yolks, olive oil and cheese in a screw-top jar. Shake very well until the dressing is completely combined. Pour over the salad leaves, toss well, and serve.

Oriental Bean Sprouts

SERVES 4

½ teaspoon ground ginger
½ small onion, very finely chopped
180ml olive oil
50ml balsamic vinegar
50ml water
2 tablespoons light soy sauce
2 teaspoons tomato ketchup
juice of ½ lemon
250g bean sprouts
1 small yellow pepper, seeded and chopped
10cm piece cucumber, cut into small dice
4 water chestnuts, thinly sliced
4 spring onions, finely chopped
1 small bunch watercress, leaves only
salt and freshly ground black pepper

Make a dressing by putting the ginger, onion, olive oil, vinegar, water, soy sauce, tomato purée and lemon juice in a screw-top jar. Shake well and season to taste. Combine the remaining ingredients in a large salad bowl and mix in as much dressing as you think it needs. Serve immediately.

Rice Salad

SERVES 4–6

basmati rice, measured up to the 250ml
   mark in a measuring jug
500ml boiling water
3 tablespoons olive oil
1 tablespoon white wine vinegar
1 small onion, very finely chopped
5cm piece cucumber, diced
3 large tomatoes, peeled and finely chopped
1 yellow pepper, seeded and finely chopped
1 eating apple, quartered, cored and chopped
50g sultanas
a few chunks of fresh or tinned pineapple, chopped
salt and freshly ground black pepper

Put the rice in a saucepan with a little salt. Add the boiling water, bring to the boil, stir, cover and leave to simmer for 15 minutes until all the water has been absorbed. Drain, if necessary, and empty the rice into a salad bowl. Make a dressing from the olive oil and white wine vinegar, and pour it over the hot rice. Allow to cool. Mix in the other ingredients, season well and serve.

A Few Simple Nut-free Salad Dressings

Classic Vinaigrette

1 teaspoon sea salt

1 garlic clove, crushed

1 teaspoon mustard powder

1 tablespoon balsamic vinegar

6 tablespoons olive oil

freshly ground black pepper

Mix together the salt, garlic, mustard and vinegar and then season well with black pepper. Put the mixture in a screw-top jar with the olive oil and shake well.

Creamy Blue Cheese Dressing

1 garlic clove, crushed

1 teaspoon sea salt

1 teaspoon Dijon mustard

2 tablespoons olive oil

1 tablespoon white wine vinegar

juice of ½ lemon

150ml crème fraîche

2 tablespoons mayonnaise

50g Danish blue

freshly ground black pepper

Mix together the garlic and the salt. Combine it with the mustard, oil, vinegar and lemon. Stir this into the crème fraîche and mayonnaise, and crumble in the Danish blue. Season with pepper.

Mustard Dressing

2 tablespoons Dijon mustard

2 tablespoons balsamic vinegar

5 tablespoons olive oil

plenty of salt and freshly ground black pepper

Put all the ingredients in a screw-top jar and shake well.

Oregano and Balsamic Dressing

2 tablespoons balsamic vinegar

5 tablespoons olive oil

4 tablespoons finely chopped fresh oregano

salt and plenty of freshly ground black pepper

Put all the ingredients in a screw-top jar and shake well.

Tangy Lemon and Lime Dressing

1 tablespoon lemon juice

1 tablespoon lime juice

1 teaspoon sea salt

plenty of freshly ground black pepper

Put all the ingredients in a screw-top jar and shake well.

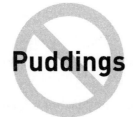

Puddings

Puddings can be a minefield for the nut-allergy sufferer. A large number of pre-prepared supermarket desserts contain nuts; and in restaurants where puddings are made there's always a chance of cross-contamination – more desserts than you would imagine contain nuts. But it doesn't mean you have to be deprived! Here are ten fabulous recipes to get your taste buds tingling, all of them completely nut-free.

Gingery Baked Peaches

SERVES 4

Note: Some almond-allergy sufferers may have a peach intolerance. Only use this recipe if you know it is safe.

4 under-ripe peaches (ripe peaches will not do for this recipe)
100ml runny honey
50g demerara sugar
3cm piece ginger, peeled and grated
100ml double cream

Preheat the oven to 190°C/Gas Mark 5. Butter a small baking dish. Peel the peaches by plunging them into boiling water. The skins should then just slip off. Halve the peaches, remove the stones, slice them and then layer them in the baking dish. Mix together the honey, sugar, ginger and cream, and pour this mixture over the peaches. Bake for about 30 minutes until golden, then serve hot.

Hot Blackcurrant Pudding

SERVES 6–8

280g plain flour
2 teaspoons baking powder
1 teaspoon salt
165g butter
140g caster sugar
1 egg
1½ teaspoons vanilla extract
175ml milk, plus a little extra for the topping
350g blackcurrants
100g demerara sugar
½ teaspoon cinnamon

Preheat the oven to 190°C/Gas Mark 5. Grease a 20cm-round baking dish.

Sift the flour, baking powder and half the salt into a dish. In a food processor combine 115g butter and the caster sugar. Mix in the egg and ½ teaspoon vanilla extract. Add the milk bit by bit until it is well combined, and then add the flour mixture spoonful by spoonful until well combined. Pour the mixture into the baking dish and sprinkle it with the blackcurrants.

Combine the demerara sugar, remaining flour, remaining salt and cinnamon. Rub in the remaining butter until it resembles coarse breadcrumbs. Sprinkle 2 tablespoons of milk and the remaining vanilla extract over the mixture and combine lightly. Sprinkle the topping over the fruit. Bake for about 45 minutes, until a skewer comes out clean.

Spicy Semolina

SERVES 4–6

1 litre full-fat milk
50g semolina
½ teaspoon salt
½ teaspoon ground ginger
½ teaspoon ground cinnamon
50g butter
250ml golden syrup
2 eggs, beaten

Preheat the oven to 180°C/Gas Mark 4. Grease a 1-litre soufflé dish.

Heat 750ml milk in a saucepan. Combine the remaining milk with the semolina, salt, ginger and cinnamon in a glass bowl. Place over a saucepan of gently simmering water, add the hot milk and stir constantly until smooth. Leave to cook for 25 minutes, stirring constantly. Remove from the heat and stir in the butter and syrup. Stir until it is all dissolved, then add the beaten eggs. Pour the mixture into the baking dish and bake for 1 hour. Serve immediately.

Chocolate Cheesecake

SERVES 10–12

80g butter

115g digestive biscuits, crushed

150g caster sugar

450g dark cooking chocolate

115g caster sugar

2 teaspoons vanilla extract

4 eggs

700g Philadelphia cheese

Preheat the oven to 170°C/Gas Mark 3. Line a 20cm cake tin with a removable base. Melt the butter and mix it with the crushed biscuits and 115g sugar. Press the mixture into the bottom of the tin. In a glass bowl set over a saucepan of simmering water melt the chocolate with the remaining sugar. Remove from the heat and stir in the vanilla extract. Leave to cool for 10 minutes. Meanwhile, combine the eggs and cream cheese, then stir in the chocolate mixture. Mix well, and pour into the cake tin. Bake for 45 minutes, leave to cool and then refrigerate overnight.

Eton Mess

SERVES 4

500g strawberries, chopped
4 tablespoons brandy
2 large egg whites
110g caster sugar
300ml double cream

Preheat the oven to 140°C/Gas Mark 1. Lightly grease a baking sheet. Put the strawberries in a bowl, sprinkle with brandy and leave to infuse while you make some meringues.

Whisk the egg whites until they are firm enough for the bowl to be held upside down without them falling out. Continue whisking and add the caster sugar a spoonful at a time. When it is all combined, use a dessertspoon to drop blobs of the mixture on to the baking sheet. Bake for 1 hour, then turn off the oven and leave till cool.

Whip the cream until soft peaks form. Fold in the strawberries. Crush the meringues into chunks, add to the strawberry and cream mixture, and fold in well. Serve immediately.

Rhubarb and Ginger Cheesecake

SERVES 6

75g butter
225g ginger biscuits, crushed (do make sure you
    buy a nut-free brand)
350g rhubarb
75g caster sugar
1 teaspoon fresh ginger, very finely chopped
3 eggs, beaten
225g Philadelphia cheese
10ml powdered gelatine
150ml double cream

Lightly grease a 20cm cake tin with a removable base. Melt the butter and stir in the biscuits. Press the mixture into the base of the cake tin. Put the rhubarb, sugar, grated ginger and a tablespoon of water in a pan, and heat very gently until the rhubarb is soft and the sugar all dissolved. Purée in a blender until smooth, then return to the pan. Beat in the eggs, and heat gently until it thickens. Do not allow it to boil or the eggs will scramble. Beat in the cheese and allow to cool. Dissolve the gelatine according to the instructions on the packet, then stir into the rhubarb mixture. Beat the cream to soft peaks, fold into the rhubarb mixture and then pour into the cake tin. Refrigerate until set.

Summer Pudding

SERVES 4–6

900g mixed summer fruits – raspberries,
    redcurrants and blackcurrants are all good
175g caster sugar
8 slices white bread

Grease a 900ml pudding basin. Prepare and rinse the fruit and put it in a saucepan with the sugar. Heat gently for about 5 minutes until the sugar has dissolved. Line the pudding basin with the slices of bread, pressing it well in. Remove a little of the juice from the fruit (you will use this to pour over the finished pudding), then pour the remaining fruit and juice into the bowl. Cover with another slice of bread. Place a saucer that just fits the top of the bowl over it, and put a heavy weight on top – a couple of bags of sugar would be good. Refrigerate overnight. Turn out on to a serving dish and serve with the reserved juice.

Nut-free Trifle

SERVES 6

6 trifle sponges – make sure they are nut-free

your favourite jam

250g fresh or frozen raspberries

50ml sherry

600ml double cream

3 egg yolks

25g caster sugar

1 teaspoon cornflour

2 bananas, finely sliced

Break up the trifle sponges into bite-sized pieces. Spread each one with a little jam, put them in a glass trifle bowl, then sprinkle the raspberries and sherry over them.

Now make the custard. Heat 300ml cream in a saucepan. In a bowl mix the egg yolks, sugar and cornflour, and pour over the hot cream, mixing well. Return it all to the saucepan and heat till thick. Leave to cool.

Mix the bananas into the custard and pour over the trifle sponges and raspberries. Whip the remaining cream and spread this over the trifle. Chill well before serving.

Chocolate Mousse

SERVES 4

200g very good-quality cooking chocolate
4 eggs, separated
3 tablespoons brandy

Place the chocolate in a glass bowl and melt it over a saucepan of simmering water. Remove from the heat and beat in the egg yolks and brandy. Leave to cool for about 10 minutes. Meanwhile, whip the cream to soft peaks and fold it into the chocolate mixture. Spoon into ramekins, cover with cling film and chill for 2 hours until firm.

Raspberry Cobbler

SERVES 6–8

750g raspberries
425g caster sugar
250g plain flour
grated rind 1 lemon
1 tablespoon baking powder
100g butter
250ml milk

Preheat the oven to 180°C/Gas Mark 4. Mix together the raspberries, 200g caster sugar, 25g plain flour and lemon rind and transfer to a 2-litre baking dish.

Sift together the remaining flour, 200g sugar and the baking powder. Melt the butter and mix with the milk. Add the milk mixture to the flour mixture bit by bit, stirring all the time until you have a smooth paste. Spoon this paste over the raspberries and spread evenly. Sprinkle the remaining sugar over the top. Bake for 50 minutes until just browned, and serve immediately.

Kids' Treats

It can be terribly difficult explaining to children that there are some things they cannot eat, even if their friends can. But, if they suffer from a nut allergy, it is the most important thing you will ever teach them. You have to be ultra careful with kids – the things that they most want to eat are often the things that put them at the biggest risk. Chocolates, sweets, cakes – they are all high-risk foods for the nut-allergy sufferer.

But this doesn't mean that your children have to feel left out. There are plenty of exciting, fun things you can make that do not present a risk to their health. Here are just a few ideas for kids' treats that will make the life of a child with a nut allergy a lot more enjoyable.

Toffee Apples

MAKES 6

6 eating apples
450g demerara sugar
150ml water
75g butter
¼ teaspoon cream of tartar
110g treacle
110g golden syrup

You will need a sugar thermometer for this recipe. Lightly grease a baking sheet. Insert a long wooden cocktail stick firmly into each apple. Put the sugar and water in a large saucepan and heat gently until the sugar is dissolved. Add the butter, cream of tartar, treacle and golden syrup, and bring to the boil. Heat to 145°C without stirring. Now dip the apples into the toffee mixture, let any excess toffee drip off, then leave to cool on the baking sheet. Eat the same day.

Gingerbread Men

MAKES 15–20

50g butter

115g caster sugar

4 tablespoons molasses

350g self-raising flour

2 teaspoons ground ginger

½ teaspoon ground cinnamon

½ teaspoon ground cloves

Preheat the oven to 180°C/Gas Mark 4. Lightly grease one or two baking sheets, depending on their size. In a food processor, beat together the butter and sugar until pale. Stir in the molasses and 3 tablespoons of water, and mix well. Sift together the remaining ingredients, add the butter and sugar mixture, and blend together until it resembles breadcrumbs. Pack the mixture together with your hands to make a soft dough. Roll out on to a lightly floured surface and cut out your gingerbread men using an appropriately shaped cutter, or a sharp knife, and transfer to the baking sheet. Bake for 10 minutes, then leave to cool on a wire rack.

Pizza

SERVES 2

For the dough:
100ml luke warm water
1 teaspoon honey
1 sachet easy-blend yeast
225g strong white flour
1 teaspoon salt
1 egg, beaten
1 teaspoon olive oil

For the topping:
1 tin tomatoes
1 teaspoon dried oregano
100g pepperoni
handful of thinly sliced mushrooms
whatever else you like on your pizza!
3 tablespoons grated Cheddar or Parmesan
salt and freshly ground black pepper

Pour 75ml of the water into a basin. Add the honey and yeast, and stir till dissolved. Place the flour and salt in a mixing bowl, pour in the yeast mixture and egg, and mix to a dough. If it seems too dry, add a little more water until you have a soft dough that does not leave any bits on the side of the bowl. Knead for about 5 minutes on a floured surface. Return to the bowl and rub with olive oil. Cover with cling film and leave in a warm place until it has doubled in size. Knead again for 3–4 minutes and then press it into a 30x25cm baking tin, pinching the edges so they raise up slightly.

Preheat the oven to 200°C/Gas Mark 7. Liquidise the tomatoes and season with the oregano, salt and pepper. Spread over the pizza base. Sprinkle over the topping ingredients, finishing with the cheese. Leave for about 10 minutes, then bake for 20 minutes until well cooked. Serve immediately with a green salad.

Fresh Fruit Jelly

SERVES 3–4

grated zest 1 orange
juice and grated zest of ½ lemon
225ml water
75g sugar
40g gelatine
450ml fresh orange juice
cream to serve

Place the orange zest, lemon juice and zest into a pan with half the water and the sugar. Heat very gently until the sugar has dissolved. Add the gelatine to the remaining water, and leave for 10 minutes. Add to the pan and heat, stirring constantly, until smooth. Strain through a sieve and allow to cool slightly before adding the orange juice and turn into serving bowls to set. Chill, then serve with the cream.

Home-made Chocolate Ice Cream

500ml milk

500ml double cream

350g sugar

20g cocoa powder

30g cooking chocolate

½ teaspoon vanilla extract

8 large egg yolks

Place the milk, cream, half the sugar, cocoa powder, chocolate and vanilla extract in a large saucepan. Heat gently, stirring, until everything is dissolved and the mixture is just simmering.

In a large bowl, beat together the eggs with the remaining sugar. Pour the hot milk over, mixing well, then transfer it all back to the pan. Heat very gently, stirring constantly until the mixture thickens. Do not overheat, as this will make the eggs curdle. Chill until cold. Pour into an ice-cream maker and churn according to the manufacturer's instructions, or alternatively pour the mixture into a Tupperware container and place in the freezer, stirring every 45 minutes until frozen.

Home-made Burgers

SERVES 4

450g very good-quality minced beef
sunflower oil for brushing
4 floury baps
thinly sliced onion
tomato ketchup
salt and freshly ground black pepper

Season the meat well with salt and pepper, and divide into four portions. Shape each portion into a ball, then press down to make a patty. Brush all over with sunflower oil, and cook under a hot grill for about 5 minutes on each side. Serve in the baps with the onions and ketchup.

Lemon Ice Cream Soda

SERVES 1

juice of ½ lemon
3 teaspoons sugar
soda water
1 large scoop vanilla ice cream

Put the lemon juice in a tall glass, add the sugar and stir until dissolved. Fill the glass about two-thirds full of soda water, then float the ice cream on top. Serve immediately with a spoon and a straw.

Orange Ice Lollies

MAKES ABOUT 5, DEPENDING ON THE SIZE OF YOUR MOULDS

100g sugar
150ml water
150ml freshly squeezed orange juice
2 tablespoons lemon juice

Combine the sugar and the water in a pan, then heat gently till dissolved. Turn up the heat and boil, without stirring, for 3 minutes. Add the orange and lemon juice, then pour into moulds and cool before freezing.

Jam Tarts

MAKES 10–12

400g plain flour
½ teaspoon salt
100g cold butter, cut into small cubes
100g cold lard, cut into small cubes
small amount of very cold water
about 12 tablespoons of your favourite jam

Sift the flour and salt into a bowl. Add the butter and lard, and rub into the flour until it resembles breadcrumbs. Add about a tablespoon of cold water and mix with a palette knife until you have a smooth dough. Add more water if you need it, but be careful not to add too much. Wrap in cling film and place in the fridge for 30 minutes. (You can make the pastry in a food processor; or you could just buy it ready-made from the supermarket – just be careful to check for nut warnings.)

Preheat the oven to 200°C/Gas Mark 6. Roll out the pastry on a floured surface, and cut out circles using a 7cm cutter. Line a bun tin with the pastry circles, then add a tablespoon of jam to the centre of each one. Place in the oven and cook for 10–15 minutes until golden. Cool on a wire rack before serving.

Chocolate Cornflake Cakes

MAKES 10–12

2 packets good-quality cooking chocolate
box of cornflakes

Melt the chocolate in a large bowl placed over a pan of boiling water. When smooth, add enough cornflakes so that they are nicely coated with chocolate, then spoon the mixture into fairy-cake cases. Leave to set, then eat!

Useful Contacts

The Anaphylaxis Campaign
PO Box 275
Farnborough
Hampshire GU14 6SX
Tel: 01252 542029
www.anaphylaxis.org.uk

Allergy UK
Deepdene House
30 Bellegrove Road
Welling
Kent DA16 3PY
Tel: 020 8303 8525
Fax: 020 8303 8792
Allergy helpline: 020 8303 8583
Email: info@allergyuk.org
www.allergyuk.org

Food Standards Agency
Aviation House
125 Kingsway
London WC2B 6NH
Tel: 020 7276 8000
Emergency helpline: 020 7270 8960
www.food.gov.uk

Food Standards Agency Scotland
St Magnus House
6th Floor
25 Guild Street
Aberdeen AB11 6NJ
Tel: 01224 285100

Food Standards Agency Wales
11th Floor
Southgate House
Wood Street
Cardiff CF10 1EW
Tel: 02920 678999

Food Standards Agency Northern Ireland
10c Clarendon Road
Belfast BT1 3BG
Tel: 02890 417700

NHS Direct Online
www.nhsdirect.nhs.uk

Allergic Reactions Central
www.allergic-reactions.com

It's Nuts Free (suppliers of nut-free products)
PO Box 380
Harrogate
North Yorkshire HG1 4XQ
Tel: 01423 561569
Fax: 01423 561572
Email: post@itsnutsfree.com
www.itsnutsfree.com

Helpful Books

Living with Nut Allergies by Karen Evennett
  (Sheldon Press)
The Kid-friendly Food Allergy Cookbook by
  Lynne Rominger and Leslie Hammond
  (Fair Winds Press)
The Allergy Bible by Linda Gamlin (Quadrille)
The Complete Guide to Food Allergy and Intolerance by
  Jonathan Brostoff and Linda Gamlin (Bloomsbury)
Change Your Diet and Change Your Life by Sharla Race
  (Bloomsbury)

Index of Recipes